BABY GIRL
or
BABY BOY

Determining the Sex of Your Child
Explained in Plain and SIMPLE Language

Mark Moore, MD and Lisa Moore, RN

Illustrated by Jeff Parker

first edition

WASHINGTON PUBLISHERS

www.washingtonpublishers.com

BABY GIRL or BABY BOY—

Determining the Sex of Your Child
Copyright 2002 by Mark Moore, MD and Lisa Moore, RN

ISBN Number 0-9715721-0-0

Washington Publishers
P.O. Box 12517, Tallahassee, Florida 32317

Publishers Cataloging-in-publication
Mark Moore, MD, Lisa Moore, RN
1. Gender pre-selection
2. Pregnancy
3. Moore, Mark
4. Moore, Lisa

ACKNOWLEDGEMENTS

To those who have helped make this book happen: your valuable assistance is greatly appreciated.

With special thanks to Wally "famous" Amos. Your kindness and generosity of spirit are exceeded only by your glowing personality. For Professor Jerry Osteryoung, his business students and their expertise. For Chip and HB. And to Jeff for your wonderful illustrations and Pat for all your review, insight and encouragement.

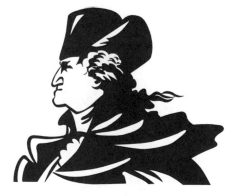

DEDICATIONS

Dedicated to our beautiful children; our family; our moms, Anita and Jerri; our dads, Paul and Donald; our brothers, Paul and Shawn; and sisters, Tahni, Roxane and Anita; Aunt Ruth and Granny; Laura, Margaret, Angela and Chris; friends near and far; friends old and new; our teachers, instructors and mentors, especially John Downs and Rafael Miguel; all the many surgeons and staff we have worked with; those who have cared for us; EJ, Steve, Katie, Mark and Melanie, Jana and Karl; counselors that have guided us; and of course, to the future mothers of our world's children.

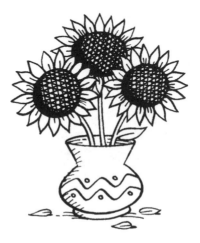

FORETHOUGHT

There is nothing more wondrous than observing the birth of a child...except, maybe, watching her or him grow up.

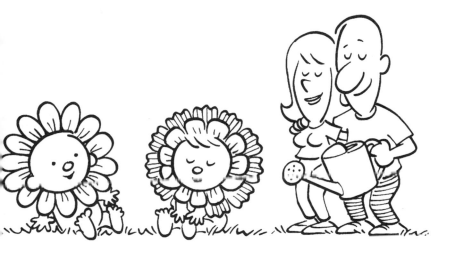

To fully understand the principles of this book, we encourage you to read each page in its entirety.

INTRODUCTION

This book is written in simple language to help future parents sway the odds of having a girl or boy. Normally it's about a 50-50 chance either way. However, when closely followed, the methods outlined in this book can improve those odds to as high as 80-20 in your favor.

The most famous person who tried to prearrange the sex of his children was King Henry VIII. After reading this, you'll agree he probably could have satisfied his desire for male heirs by simply monitoring his bedchamber activities!

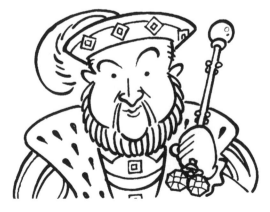

TABLE OF CONTENTS

pg.

THE MAN

The man has TESTES (also called testicles), which make and store the SPERM.

These testes live in the external SCROTAL SAC (SCROTUM) to control the proper temperature for sperm production, which is slightly cooler than the body's normal temperature of 98.6 degrees Fahrenheit.

TESTOSTERONE is a male hormone made by the testes, which assists in the production and growth of the sperm.

During sex, the man ejaculates about 1/8 ounce of semen, containing approximately 300,000 sperm.

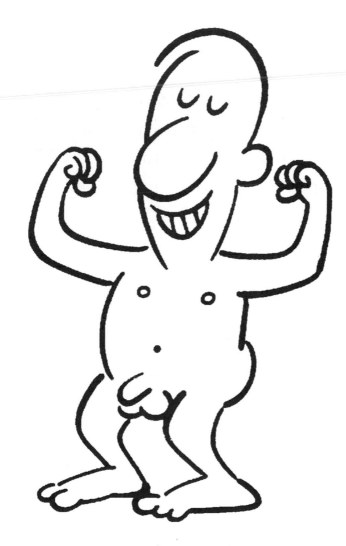

THE SPERM

The man produces two kinds of sperm: X-SPERM and Y-SPERM. During conception, one of these unites with the woman's egg and determines the baby's gender (BABY GIRL when the X-Sperm unites with the egg or BABY BOY when the Y-Sperm unites with the egg). The two types of sperm have different characteristics as described below:

X-SPERM traits:
oval heads, move slower, live longer,
much stronger, far fewer X-Sperm than Y-Sperm

Y-SPERM traits:
round heads, move faster, die faster, more fragile,
many more Y-sperm than X-sperm

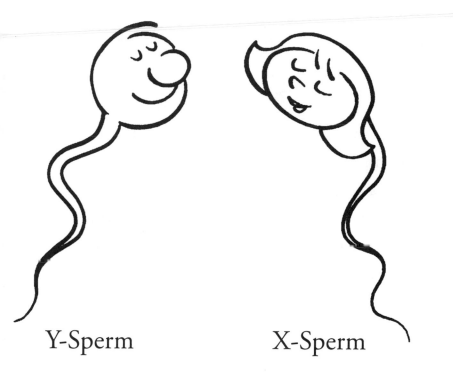

Y-Sperm   X-Sperm

THE WOMAN

The woman has two OVARIES and a UTERUS
(WOMB). The EGG grows in either of the
ovaries with the influence of female hormones
such as estrogen.

One time per monthly cycle, an egg bursts out
from an ovary (OVULATION) and travels down
the FALLOPIAN TUBES into the uterus.
If it happens to unite with the sperm there
(CONCEPTION), the egg then implants itself,
creating a new entity called a ZYGOTE. This
represents the beginning of an extraordinary
process—the development of your future baby.

As an additional note, when a female reaches
orgasm, her body produces an emission of alkaline
fluids. This can actually help the Y-Sperm if it
occurs BEFORE the male ejaculation.

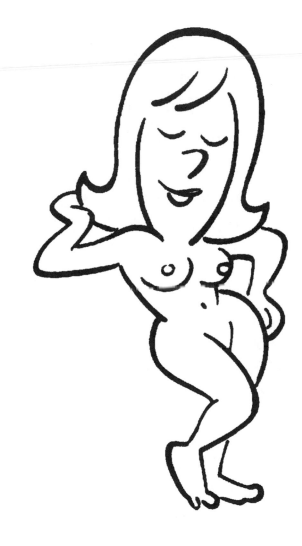

THE EGG

The woman produces only one type of EGG—the X-Egg. Sometimes multiple eggs burst out, and if each one becomes fertilized by the sperm, multiple births such as twins or triplets can result. In these cases, each fertilized egg will create individually unique FRATERNAL siblings. Sometimes one fertilized egg splits once or more, creating exact duplicate babies, known as IDENTICAL twins, triplets, etc.

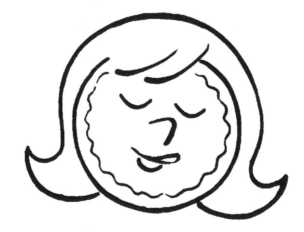

THE CYCLE

The female monthly CYCLE is extremely important in determining the OVULATION DATE. Typically, the average cycle is 28 days, although normal variation and irregularity sometimes occur— even in the same female. Under the influence of female hormones such as estrogen, the lining of the uterus grows to prepare for the possibility of egg fertilization. Should this not occur during a cycle, the uterine lining disintegrates and discharges as menstrual flow.

- Day 1 is the first day of bleeding
- Bleeding usually lasts from Day 1 through Day 5
- Day 14 is typically ovulation time in a consistent 28-day cycle, but this can vary

Ideally, the female should track her BASAL BODY TEMPERATURE for two months on a paper graph. It's best to do this every morning before getting out of bed (details on page 28).

Usually, ovulation corresponds to a day on the graph when the woman's body temperature falls slightly and then suddenly rises by at least a degree Fahrenheit. Some women may feel an abdominal "tingle" around the time when the egg "bursts" out, corresponding to a surge in hormone levels. Specific ovulation kits, which can measure these hormone peaks, are available in your local pharmacy and can be quite accurate.

THE CONCEPTION

There are only three possible players in this game:

1. Egg (X)
2. Sperm (X)
3. Sperm (Y)

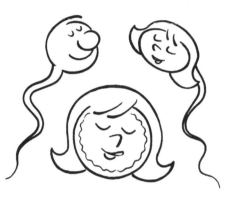

With two possible results:

1. X-egg and X-sperm make XX (baby girl)
2. X-egg and Y-sperm make XY (baby boy)

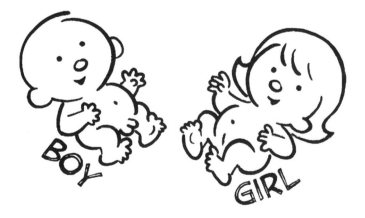

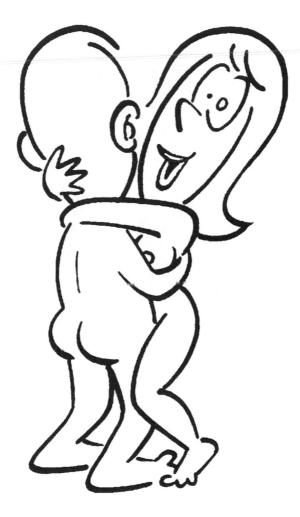

TRYING FOR A BABY BOY

You want the Y-SPERM to be more plentiful and make its way to the EGG easier and faster. That's why you must first determine your OVULATION DATE, and avoid sexual intercourse and activity at certain times to build up the sperm count.

For alkaline douche and dietary influences, see page 25.

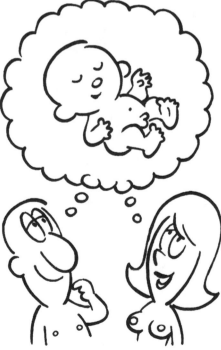

INCREASE YOUR CHANCES OF HAVING A
BABY BOY:

1. No intercourse (or anything else) for 3 to 4 days before the calculated OVULATION DATE. This will help increase the sperm count.
2. No hot tubs, baths or briefs for the man for at least one week prior.
3. Have intercourse ONE TIME ONLY on the OVULATION DATE, and use condoms for any sex during the next 2 to 3 days.
4. Ideally, the woman should reach orgasm before the man.
5. Enjoy long foreplay and sexual excitement to maximize sperm emission.
6. The male should enter the female from behind ("doggie-style")
7. At climax, the man should deposit deeply.
8. The man should drink coffee or caffeinated soda 2 hours before sex, which can increase sperm counts.
9. After sex, sperm retention is improved if the female lies still for 20 minutes.
10. Avoid artificial lubricants during sex.

TRYING FOR A BABY GIRL

You want the X-SPERM to be more plentiful in this case. Determine the OVULATION DATE. Because the X-Sperm live longer, you should have sexual intercourse 3 days BEFORE your calculated OVULATION DATE. This means that mostly X-Sperm will survive to fertilize the egg 3 days later.

For acidic vinegar douche and dietary influences, see page 25.

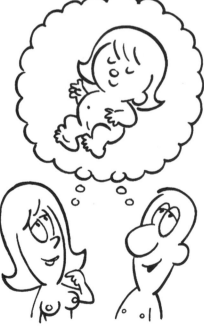

INCREASE YOUR CHANCES OF HAVING A
BABY GIRL:

For discussion purposes, let's use an ovulation date of Day 14.

1. In order to lower the sperm count, have *frequent* intercourse on Days 5 through 8 of your cycle. This means mostly X-Sperm will prevail.
2. On Days 9,10 and 11, have *daily* intercourse using the methods described below.
3. The sexual position should be face-to-face.
4. Keep foreplay or excitement to a minimum.
5. During the man's climax, he should pull back and deposit shallow.
6. Avoid artificial lubricants during sex.
7. No sex on Days 12,13 or 14, and for at least 2 days after ovulation date, unless the man uses condoms.
8. The mini-calendar below can be used as a guide.

Sun	Mon	Tue	Wed	Thur	Fri	Sat
	◄— FREQUENT SEX TO LOWER SPERM COUNT —►				YES!	YES!
YES!	No Sex	No Sex	**OD** No Sex	No Sex	No Sex	

YES! = Have sex on these days using the methods described on this page.
OD = Ovulation Date
No Sex = No unprotected sexual intercourse; use condoms.

EITHER WAY, IT SHOULD BE FUN TRYING

- Strengthening your relationship.
- Trying new things.
- Having more sex.
- Discussing stuff.

So "go forth and multiply," and remember, each child is a gift to his or her family and the world no matter what the gender.

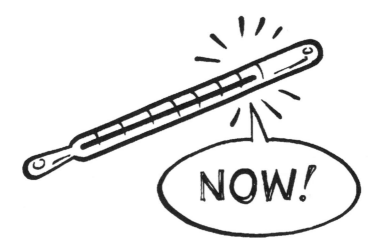

NOW!

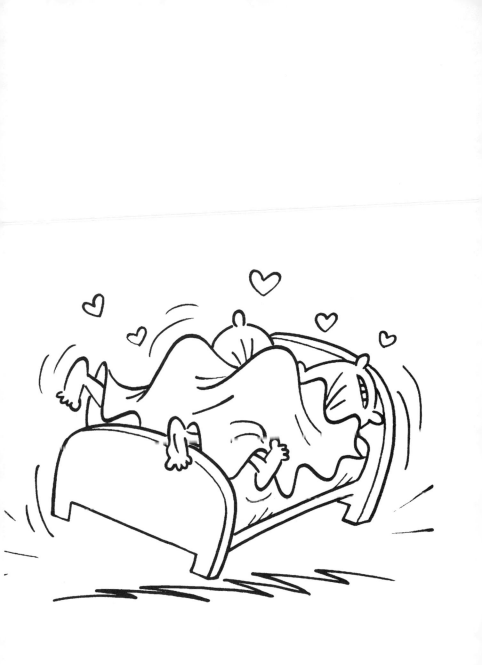

PREGNANCY POINTERS

Choose healthy foods; take your vitamins and folic acid.
Avoid alcohol, cigarettes, drugs and stress.
See your obstetrician or midwife regularly.
Read a good book on pregnancy.
Avoid gaining too much weight.

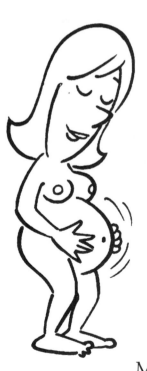

Breast feed for 6 months—it's good for baby and mama; then consider using a high-quality formula (in place of whole milk) within their diet until sixteen to eighteen months. If you have a video camera, tape 60 seconds of video and audio each week, beginning with the last 3 months of pregnancy and continuing on for several years. Watch this video journal every year on your child's birthday. Make the most of the early years because your little ones will grow up fast.

MISCELLANEOUS

WARNING! Before using any douche (which can alter vaginal secretions) or changing your diet, you must CONSULT YOUR OB/GYN, PHYSICIAN OR MIDWIFE.

Alkaline douche prior to sex (may favor Baby Boy):
add 2 tablespoonfuls of baking soda to 1 cup of sterilized water (boiled then cooled to room temp before use), and mix in sterilized douche bottle. Make within 2 hours of use.

Acidic/vinegar douche prior to sex (may favor Baby Girl):
add 2 tablespoonfuls of vinegar to a quart of sterilized water and mix in sterilized douche bottle. Make within 2 hours of use.

Mother-to-be's diet high in sodium and potassium, including vegetables, meats, salt (caution), fish, bananas and chocolate (not too much!) for the month before trying may favor Baby Boy.

Mother-to-be's diet high in calcium and magnesium, like milk, cheese, cereals, beans and nuts for the month before trying may favor a Baby Girl.

*Dietary factors have less influence on the baby's gender than other factors described in this book. A good general rule is to eat a healthy diet during the time you are trying to get pregnant.

MYTHS
about carrying your baby once you are pregnant

If the baby's heartrate is FAST, it's a girl;
   if SLOW, it's a boy.

If the mother craves SWEETS, it's a girl;
   mother craves SOUR, it's a boy.

If the mother carries HIGH, it's a girl;
   carries LOW, a boy.

If the mother is SLEEPY, it will be a girl;
   ENERGETIC mom, a boy.

If the baby kicks LOW in the belly, it's a girl;
    if kicks HIGH in the ribs, a boy.

If mother likes to sleep on her RIGHT side, a girl;
    mother sleeps on the LEFT side, a boy.

If grandma has COLORED hair, it will be a girl;
    if she has GREY hair, it will be a boy.

If mother carries SIDEWAYS, it will be a girl;
    if carries in FRONT, it will be a boy.

SAMPLE OVULATION CHART

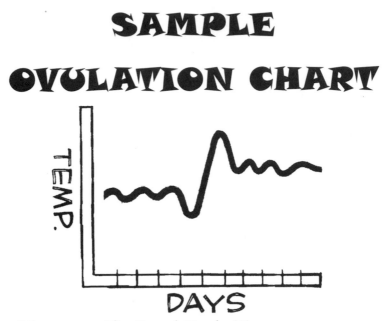

1. Use a specific Basal Body Temperature thermometer available in your local pharmacy. It includes a blank chart for daily recording.
2. Measure temperature at the same time each morning before arising, and record for 2 months.
3. The OVULATION DATE (OD) occurs when there is a slight temperature drop followed by a sudden rise in temperature (a degree or more). See sample graph above.
4. Most commonly, the ovulation date will be 14 days prior to the beginning of your next cycle. For example: 28-Day cycle, OD is Day 14 (28-14=14); on a 34-Day cycle, OD is Day 20 (34-14=20).
5. Also note there is an increase in the amount and slipperiness of vaginal mucus at ovulation date.

DISCLAIMER

The authors and publisher specifically disclaim any responsibility or any liability for loss or risk, personal or otherwise, which is incurred directly or indirectly from the use and application of any of the contents within this book. While simplified for our readers into an easy-to-read text, there is an enormous variety of conclusions and opinions within this subject matter. We assume no liability for errors, omissions or differences of opinion. Its authors are not engaged in rendering professional services or medical advice in the context of this book.

If you are having difficulty getting pregnant, then you should NOT do anything that might lower sperm counts as it could also lessen your chances of becoming pregnant, too. Sperm counts can be temporarily lowered when using the techniques of "trying for a baby girl." If you have irregular monthly cycles, it may be difficult to fulfill the details described in "trying for a baby girl" as your ovulation date may occur earlier than expected.

As always, consult your obstetrician, physician or midwife.

AFTERWORD

This book is most effective when reviewed several times, preferably with your spouse or partner.

Once you've made the decision to bring a baby into your world, you've embraced life in an entirely new light. While this book was designed to help you make the most of methods that could possibly determine your baby's gender, each infant represents a gift—whether a girl or boy.

Nothing can compare to the miracle of life—the cry of your newborn drawing the first breath or the innocence of this new baby cradled in your arms.

That's why it is so important to read everything you can about your pregnancy and become familiar with the changes that occur in your body and the expectations of future parenthood. Be generous with your time and love.

For a list of resources and suggested reading, please visit us at www.washingtonpublishers.com

AB OUT THE AUTHORS

Mark Moore, MD, is a husband, father, writer, inventor and teacher. He is a Diplomate of the American Board of Anesthesiology and board-certified in pain management, with subspecialties in obstetric and pediatric anesthesia.

Lisa Moore, RN, his wife, is a mother and a pediatric nurse. Together they have a girl, a boy, a dog and a bird.

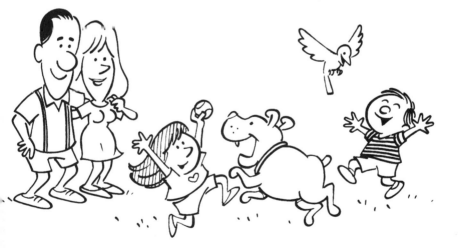

BABY GIRL or BABY BOY ORDER FORM

Fastest: ONLINE ORDERS:
www.washingtonpublishers.com

or: FAX ORDERS: 850-222-2222

MAIL ORDERS:
Washington Publishers
P.O. Box 12517, Tallahassee, FL 32317

TOLL-FREE PHONE ORDERS: 1-866-447-5269
(1-866-GIRLBOY)

ALL ORDERS MUST INCLUDE PAYMENT.

PAYMENT BY MONEY ORDER OR
CREDIT CARD FOR FASTEST SERVICE

$12.95   PER BOOK

$ 6.95   SHIPPING AND HANDLING

TOTAL: **$ 19.90**

Name_____

Address _____

City _____ State _____ Zip_____

Phone: _____ Email _____

VISA   MC   # _____

EXP. DATE _____ / _____

Special prices on bulk orders available for physicians' offices
Send email query to info@washingtonpublishers.com